Travel-Friendly Fitness

Exercise and Nutrition Tips for Jetsetters

Table of Contents

Chapter 1. Introduction

Discover a revolution in travel wellness through our Special Report on "Travel-Friendly Fitness: Exercise and Nutrition Tips for Jetsetters." This power-packed guide ensures no destination disturbs your diet or deters your fitness routine. Imagine being on that long-awaited trip and not worrying about skipping workouts or compromising on your diet. Sounds amazing, right? Curl up comfortably and delve into expert advice, age-old secrets, and modern methodologies that blend seamlessly with your journey. Our Special Report is your trusted companion, ensuring your health doesn't need a vacation while you're on one! Inspiring, achievable, and surprisingly fun - it's time to make every trip a journey towards optimal fitness. Buckle up, jetsetters, this Special Report turns 'travel fit' from whimsical wish to a no-compromise reality!

Chapter 2. Understanding Travel and Fitness: The New Norm

Preparing for a trip awakens a range of emotions - excitement, anticipation, and for those diligent about their health and fitness, a dose of apprehension. However, in recent years, a new narrative has begun to unfold in the global realm of travel, one that combines the pleasure of exploring new places with maintaining good health and fitness. This paradigm shift is reshaping the behavior of transient guests, turning even the most nomadic traveler into a health-conscious jetsetter.

2.1. Prepping Mind and Body for the Journey

Before embarking on your adventure, it's essential to prepare both your body and mind. To start with, understand that maintaining fitness requires more than sporadic physical activity. It's a holistic approach that encompasses exercise, proper nutrition, mental well-being, and adequate rest.

1. **Get Doctor's Clearance:** If you're planning to incorporate an exercise regimen into your travel, consult your medical professional before you decide on a program. Ensure that it's suitable for your physical condition and won't cause any adverse health effects.

2. **Set Realistic Goals:** Keep your fitness goals achievable, and don't let travel be an excuse for backsliding. But, maintain a balanced perspective. Understand that while travel might alter your routine, any physical activity is better than none.

3. **Stay Positive:** Adopt a positive mindset towards fitness. Believe that you can stay fit while traveling, and you'll find half the battle is already won. Taking along a motivational book or having a few inspirational quotes at hand can help reinforce your commitment to your health.

2.2. Exercise Strategies for Continuous Travel

Staying fit requires deliberate action, and this doesn't change simply because you're traveling. On the contrary, traveling offers new opportunities to imbibe a diverse range of exercise regimes—here are a few strategies that can help you maintain your fitness momentum.

1. **Hotel Workouts:** Pick hotels equipped with a gym or fitness center, and factor in a short workout session every day. If it's not possible, perform bodyweight exercises in your room. Every bit counts!

2. **Walk, Bike, and Swim:** Walking, cycling, swimming, hiking - these are all activities that ignite the joy of exploration while keeping you fit. Choose sightseeing options that let you have the best of both worlds.

3. **Stretching and Yoga:** Easily accomplished within the confines of your hotel room or even an airport waiting lounge, stretching and yoga positions can help counteract the discomfort experienced during long flights or car trips.

2.3. Roadmap to Nutritional Balance

While fine dining and exotic local foods are a part of the travel allure, maintaining a nutritional balance is equally, if not more, important. Here are a few tips to adhere to while traveling:

1. **Stay Hydrated:** Hydration is vital, especially while traveling. Drink plenty of water and avoid alcoholic and caffeinated beverages on flights as they dehydrate your body.

2. **Eat Small, Frequent Meals:** Instead of starving yourself for that big dinner, snack healthily throughout the day. This fights off cravings and keeps your metabolism running smoothly.

3. **Incorporate Protein:** Keep your protein intake high. If local cuisine is less plentiful on protein, enrich your meals with protein bars.

2.4. Technology: Your Fitness Ally

Leverage the power of technology to sustain your health and fitness. Fitness apps, wearable devices, and even social media networks act as a supplement to your fitness routine.

1. **Fitness Apps:** With guided workouts, meal plans, and motivational tips, fitness apps act as personal trainers. MyFitnessPal, Nike Training Club, and Strava are a few popular choices.

2. **Wearable Tech:** Devices like Fitbit or Apple Watch can track your physical activity, heart rate, and even sleep patterns, providing insights into your health.

3. **Social Media:** Following fitness influencers or joining fitness groups on social networks can offer encouragement and keep you updated on the latest workout trends.

By integrating these strategies seamlessly into your travel routine, health and wellness need not be compromised. As you traverse through unfamiliar terrains, savour unique cuisines, and interact with diverse cultures, remember: fitness travel has become the norm. It is an island that you carry with you, an abode of strength and vitality that leads to essential self-discovery. Fitness allows you to explore life's remarkable journey without neglecting the most important journey – towards a healthier you.

Chapter 3. Conscious Eating: Nutritional Strategies for Travelers

Navigating culinary options while on the go can be a challenge, especially when attempting to maintain a healthy diet. However, with a little guidance and careful planning, eating healthfully while travelling doesn't need to be a daunting task. The key is to learn how to balance enjoyment and nutrition – mastering the art of 'conscious eating.'

3.1. Pre-Travel Preparation

The first stage on the path to conscious eating is preparing effectively before your travels begin. It's essential to research your destination's food culture and plan around dietary restrictions if necessary. Familiarizing with local cuisines, finding suitable restaurants, and making arrangements for special dietary considerations will not only save time but can also lessen stress and anxiety.

Select a hotel with a kitchenette so that you can prepare some of your meals, and be sure to pack healthy travel snacks. These can range from dried fruit and nuts to protein bars or granola, offering key nutrients to keep your energy levels up during long travel days.

Consider bringing a reusable water bottle to ensure you stay hydrated, which is critical for digestion and overall health. If possible, also take small portions of whole-grain cereals, oatmeal, and other non-perishable foods.

3.2. Eating Out without Ditching Health Goals

For a traveler, exploring local restaurants and eateries is an integral part of the travel experience. However, it can often result in consuming excess calories and unhealthy ingredients. The solution? Making smart choices.

When ordering, check for the healthiest options on the menu – such as grilled, steamed, or roasted foods. Avoid anything fried, breaded, or described as creamy or buttery, to reduce calorie intake. Remember to stay mindful of portion sizes, which are often larger in restaurants.

Another strategy is to fill half your plate with vegetables as a rule of thumb. You'll still have room to taste other local fare while ensuring you're meeting your nutrient requirements.

3.3. Balancing Indulgences

Traveling is a time to relax, unwind, and sometimes indulge. Accepting that an occasional treat won't completely derail your nutrition goals is important, while also understanding the need for moderation.

The key lies in making conscious choices. If you choose to try a rich, local dessert, reduce or avoid added sugars for the rest of the day.

If you plan on enjoying a high-calorie meal, balance it out with lighter, nutrient-rich meals throughout the remainder of the day, with a focus on lean proteins, fruits, and vegetables.

3.4. Managing Jet Lag and Nutrition

Long-haul flights can disrupt your body's circadian rhythms leading to jet lag, which may impact your diet. Combat this by eating lean proteins and vegetables during the flight, and avoid consuming alcohol which can exacerbate dehydration and fatigue.

Once you've arrived, try to adapt immediately to the new time zone's eating schedule. This helps to realign your body clock, reducing jet lag symptoms.

3.5. Supplementing Wisely

While whole foods should be the primary source of nutrients, sometimes circumstances may call for supplements. Sometimes it may be tricky to get certain essential nutrients while traveling, such as fiber, probiotics, and certain vitamins.

Carry a supply of reliable multi-vitamins and consider a quality probiotic to aid digestion, particularly if traveling to a destination with different food hygiene standards.

3.6. Staying Hydrated

Staying hydrated while traveling is vital. Drinking plenty of water aids digestion, keeps your skin glowing, and prevents fatigue. However, when visiting countries with questionable tap water, only drink bottled or purified water to avoid potential health risks.

3.7. Mindful Eating: En Route to Conscious Eating

Conscious eating is not solely about making the right food choices but also involves eating mindfully. Mindful eating centers around paying attention to the experience of eating, listening to hunger and fullness cues, and savoring and appreciating the food you eat.

When you eat mindfully, you are more likely to make healthier food choices, enjoy your food more, and stop eating once you're satiated, rather than stuffed.

The road to nutritional wellness begins with conscious decision-making. Traveling does not have to be a roadblock on your wellness journey, but rather an opportunity to explore and instill better habits, refining your relationship with food in the process. So gear up and prepare for a nutritional adventure, because health and wellness are potentially the best souvenirs you can bring back from your travel escapades.

Chapter 4. Exercise On-the-Go: Compact and Efficient Travel Workouts

Traveling doesn't have to mean skipping your daily workout routine. While challenging, maintaining a fitness regime on-the-go is not only possible but can also be an exciting twist to your regular routine. That's where the concept of compact and efficient workouts comes into play. These workouts require minimal equipment, time, and space but ensure maximum results. Let's delve deeper into understanding how to remain physically active even while jet-setting around the globe.

4.1. Gearing up for Fitness-on-the-fly

Prepare yourself for fitness-on-the-fly by packing the right gear. Start with workout clothes that are lightweight and easy-to-pack. A dry-fit, sweat-wicking shirt teamed with a pair of shorts makes for an ideal travel-friendly gym outfit. Don't forget comfortable gym shoes or sports sneakers.

For efficient space utilization, consider multi-purpose clothing like sports bras for women that can double as swimwear, or dry-fit shirts that can be used for both workouts and a casual stroll in the city. Pack resistance bands, a jump rope, and a foldable yoga mat - these are lightweight tools that pack flat and can facilitate a variety of exercises.

4.2. The Art of Utilizing the Environment

The environment you're in can be a surprising catalyst for your workout sessions. Whether you're in a hotel room, at a beach, or amidst nature, each space has something to offer.

If you're in a hotel room, you can use the furniture for various exercises. Chair squats, elevated push-ups on the bed, and tricep dips on the coffee table, are examples of how everyday objects can be workout equipment.

When at a beach, indulge in swimming, beach volleyball, or simply jogging. The resistance of the sand to your feet acts as an excellent muscle toner. Moreover, workouts in the natural environment always bring an additional mood-enhancing benefit.

Public parks, usually equipped with benches and open spaces, can be excellent spots for performing exercises like step-ups, push-ups, and a variety of bodyweight exercises.

4.3. Setting the Pace: High-Intensity Interval Training (HIIT)

The essence of travel-friendly workouts is to maximize efficiency - gaining the most out of limited time and space. High-Intensity Interval Training fulfils this criterion perfectly. HIIT workouts involve quick and hard bursts of exercises, followed by short recovery periods. This amplifies your heart rate, leading to heavy calorie expenditure in a short 20-30 minute workout.

Incorporate exercises like jump squats, mountain climbers, plyometric lunges, and high knees. Mix and match these, perform each for about 45 seconds with a 15 second rest period, and repeat for desired rounds.

4.4. Power of Body Weight Workouts

Bodyweight workouts rely on your own body mass for resistance. Since they don't require any equipment, they are extremely travel-friendly. Exercises such as push-ups, sit-ups, lunges, planks, squats, and burpees are all examples of bodyweight exercises.

Depending on your fitness levels, these can be modified, for instance, push-ups from the knees if you're a beginner rather than full push-ups, or single-leg squats for advanced levels. These exercises work multiple muscle groups, helping you maintain strength and flexibility.

4.5. Yoga and Stretching Essentials

Yoga can be performed anywhere, and the yoga mat you've packed will come in handy here. Incorporate sequences like the Sun Salutations (Surya Namaskar), which includes a series of twelve powerful yoga poses with profound benefits. Apart from its physical benefits like improving strength, flexibility, and posture, yoga also helps in relaxation and stress reduction, which often accompanies travel.

End each workout session with a 10-minute stretching routine to cool down and loosen your muscles. This will enhance flexibility, reduce soreness, and help in muscle recovery, preparing you for your next exciting travel day.

4.6. Sticking to the Plan

While incorporating these travel workouts seems compelling, staying consistent is crucial. Dedicate a specific time slot for your workout and treat it as any other important appointment. Overcome excuses by remembering the endorphins rush post-workout and the sense of achievement it offers.

Try these compact, and efficient travel workouts, and ensure your fitness regime sails smoothly through any travels. With a little determination and creativity, your jet-setting lifestyle need not impact your fitness journey. You can enjoy your travels without any fitness compromises, truly bringing "Travel Friendly Fitness" to life!

Chapter 5. Healthy Habits: Fitness Rituals for Every Time Zone

Adopting and integrating a robust fitness routine in your daily life can be challenging, especially when you are on the move and constantly switching time zones. This challenge can seem daunting initially but with the right planning, discipline, and mindset you can overcome these hurdles. Here is a comprehensive guide on the best strategies to maintain your fitness routine while you traverse time zones.

5.1. Keeping Up with Jet Lag

Jet lag is perhaps one of the biggest challenges for travelers who frequently hop between time zones. It can affect your mood, physical performance, mental clarity, and overall disrupt your fitness routine. Let's delve into implementing different strategies to combat this transient disorder.

1. Stick to your fitness routine: Try to maintain your workout routine as best as you can irrespective of the time zone differences. This can help reset your body clock to deal with jet lag faster. If you usually work out in the morning in your home town, work out in the morning at your destination.

2. Adopt a Proper Sleeping Schedule: Getting quality sleep significantly impacts your performance and productivity. In order to adjust quickly to a new time zone, try to adapt to the local bedtime as soon as you can.

3. Hydration is the Key: Drink plenty of water before, during, and after your flight to reduce the effects of dehydration due to air travel. Water-rich fruits and vegetables can be a good option for a

nutritious boost.

5.2. Adapting Your Nutrition Plan

When you change time zones, not only do you need to tweak your workout plan, but also your eating habits. Master the art of eating well while traveling, and you can stay on track with your fitness goals as well.

1. Pack Snacks for the Process: Engage your time in the air by consuming small, nutrient-dense snacks at your typical mealtimes according to your home time zone. Nuts, fresh fruits, and protein bars can satiate your hunger.

2. Adapt Gradually: After reaching your new schedule, try to match your meals to the local times. Eat light for the first few days, helping your digestion adjust to the new schedule.

3. Stock up on Local Produce: Once reaching your destination, purchasing local fruits and vegetables helps ensure you're getting nutrients- and it's a fun way to explore local produce markets!

5.3. Designing Flexible Workout Schedules

A flexible workout routine is a savior for frequent travelers. Instead of sticking to rigid schedules, crafting versatile fitness rituals can be more suitable and realistic.

1. Embrace Body-Weight Exercises: Body-weight exercises like push-ups, lunges, squats, jumping jacks, and planks can be done anywhere. Incorporate these into your routine to stay fit without needing any equipment.

2. Walking or Cycling for Sightseeing: Opt to walk or cycle while exploring a new city. This is an excellent strategy to keep you

active and also a great way to experience new surroundings more intimately.

3. Online Fitness Classes: The modern tech-savvy world brings fitness classes to your fingertips. Whether it's yoga, high-intensity interval training (HIIT workouts), or Pilates, find an online class that fits into your schedule.

5.4. Ensuring Mental Wellness

Fitness doesn't solely rely on physical activity and nutrition. Mental wellness plays an equally crucial role in your overall well-being. While changing time zones, paying attention to your mental health is important.

1. Practice Mindfulness: Whether it's through meditation, deep breathing exercises or simply enjoying a quiet moment in a park, mindfulness practices can significantly alleviate stress and promote a positive mood.

2. Maintain Social Connection: Cultivating and maintaining connections with people, reaching out to family and friends, or making new acquaintances can significantly uplift your mood.

3. Digital Detox: While technology can be a valuable tool in maintaining fitness, it's also important to disconnect from our digital devices from time to time. Regular digital detox can improve your sleep and reduce anxiety.

5.5. Embracing the Local Lifestyle

Understanding and integrating into the local lifestyle can be a game-changer in maintaining your fitness routine. The key to this approach lies in keeping an open mind and a willingness to adapt to change.

1. Learn from the Locals: Whether that's practicing Tai Chi in a park in China or eating sushi in Japan, integrating local health rituals

can enhance fitness journey on the go.

2. Local Sports: Participating in local sports activities can be a great strategy to get moving, and it allows for cultural immersion. It might be a friendly game of beach volleyball at Copacabana or a simple table tennis match with locals in Berlin.

This ultimate travel fitness guide addresses the challenges posed by different time zones and empowers you to stay in shape, maintain your workout routine, keep up with a healthy diet, and above all, enjoy the journey as you traverse the world. Whether it's acclimating to jet lag, maintaining your nutrition, setting up flexible work routines, fostering mental wellness, or embracing local lifestyles, this guide offers you the tools to seamlessly integrate fitness into your travel rituals without compromising on your exploration and experience. Now the world becomes not just your playground, but your fitness studio as well.

Chapter 6. Fitpacking: Smart Selection and Packing of Fitness Gear

Traveling is an adventure, a chance to explore new cultures, learn new languages, and taste new cuisines. Yet, for fitness enthusiasts, it also presents a challenge: how to maintain a healthy lifestyle while on the move. One of the most crucial components of fitness-friendly travel is the savvy selection and smart packing of your fitness gears. Let's look upon it in a detailed manner.

6.1. Choosing the Right Fitness Gear

When choosing the right fitness gears, there are three key factors to consider: portability, versatility, and necessity.

Portable fitness equipment should be compact, lightweight, and easy to pack. These could include resistance bands, jump ropes, and portable suspension trainers. Resistance bands, for example, are an incredible multi-purpose tool. They're lightweight, affordable, and can provide a full-body workout with minimal space requirements.

Versatile fitness equipment can adapt to a variety of workout routines. For example, a yoga mat can serve as a base for pilates, stretching, meditation, and bodyweight exercises. Similarly, suspension trainers are excellent tools for strength training, balance, and flexibility exercises.

The necessity refers to fitness tools that you use regularly and are crucial for maintaining your fitness routine. These could be running shoes for the avid runner or a swimming cap and goggles for a water workout enthusiast.

Remember, everyone's fitness needs and requirements are different, so what works for one person might not work for another. Compile a list of the fitness gears that you frequently use and prioritize them based on their portability and versatility.

6.2. Pack like a Pro

Knowing what to pack is just half the battle; the real game is in packing all of your fitness equipment efficiently without adding unnecessary weight or bulk to your luggage. Here are some expert tips:

1. Utilize Every Space: Shoes make a great storage area for small items like socks or resistance bands. Remember to put these items in a bag to avoid any dirt or smell touching the rest of your items.

2. Roll, Don't Fold: Rolling clothes can free up space for other items. You can roll your workout clothes and put them inside your shoes or any other gaps.

3. Vacuum Seal Bags: If space is at a premium and you wish to carry bulky items like a yoga mat or foam roller, consider using vacuum seal bags. They can reduce the volume of these items significantly.

4. Place heavy items towards the bottom: This helps maintain the balance of your bag, avoiding any top-heavy scenarios where your bag could topple over.

6.3. Maintenance and Care of the Fitness Gear

While on the move, maintaining your fitness gear is essential to ensure it lasts and performs well. Rinse your workout clothes after a session, as leaving them damp can lead to unpleasant odours. Most resistance bands can be wiped clean with a damp cloth. Let them air dry, avoid exposure to direct sunlight, which can degrade the material

6.4. When Fitness Gear Isn't Accessible

There will be times when notwithstanding your best packing efforts, you simply can't carry all the gear you would like. For such scenarios, it's important to be resourceful and adaptable. Familiarize yourself with bodyweight exercises and yoga poses, which rely on the body's weight for resistance and can be done anywhere.

6.5. The Future of Travel-Friendly Fitness Gear

Innovation never stops, and fitness gear is no exception. Companies are continuously developing compact, lightweight, and portable fitness equipments that can be easily packed and carried wherever we go. Smart ropes, foldable weights, compact sliders for core workouts are some of the tools that we could expect in the coming years.

In conclusion, the right selection and packing of fitness gear can make a world of difference in maintaining your fitness routine while traveling. With the right strategies in place, you can ensure that no travel and adventure can distract you from your path to fitness. It's all about preparation, planning, and the willingness to remain flexible and adapt. After all, fitness is as much a journey as it is a destination.

Chapter 7. Menu Matters: How to Eat Healthy, Anywhere, Anytime

Dining out while traveling is an exciting opportunity to indulge in the exotic, foreign flavors that each unique destination presents. Yet, these gastronomic adventures shouldn't derail your ongoing commitment to healthy eating. This comprehensive guide provides practical strategies for making wise food choices anytime, anywhere.

7.1. Deciphering the Menu

Not all menus are created equal. Many tend to lean towards offering dishes that are high in fats, sugars, and salts. The key is to decipher them, finding balance between health and indulgence.

When reading the menu, look for words such as "grilled," "steamed," "roasted," or "baked." These preparations usually involve fewer fats. Conversely, items described as "fried," "battered," "breaded," or "creamy" are more likely to be high in unhealthy fats and calories.

Ask questions about the preparation methods to ensure you're making informed choices. Most restaurants will be more than happy to accommodate special dietary requests. You can often ask for sauces on the side, less oil, or extra vegetables, for instance.

Typically, a sizable portion of restaurant meals consist of carbs. You can balance this by ordering an additional side of veggies, asking for a double portion of protein, or even replacing the starch component altogether with a healthier alternative if available.

7.2. Eating in Portions

Portion control is, without a doubt, one of the most crucial elements of eating healthy on the go. Here's how to manage your portion sizes when dining out:

1. Divide your plate: Imagine your plate divided into four quarters. Half of your plate should contain veggies, a quarter for lean protein, and the remaining quarter for carbs, preferably whole grains.

2. Practice mindful eating: Pay attention to the food that's on your plate. Savor each bite, eating slowly, and chewing thoroughly. This practice aids digestion and also promotes a sense of fullness.

3. Beware of starters and sides: Many starters and sides are a hidden source of extra calories. Choose wisely or opt to skip this part of the meal altogether.

4. Engage in conversation: Distracting yourself by talking to your dining partners can help slow your eating pace, allowing your brain to recognize when you're full.

7.3. On-board Airplane Meals and Snacks

Airplane food is notorious for its high salt and low nutrient content. The pressure and dry air inside the aircraft cabin can alter taste perception, making food taste bland, thus the overuse of salt and spices.

In this scenario, ordering a special low-sodium or vegetarian meal prior to your flight can be a good option. If available, opt for fresh fruits or yogurt for refreshments instead.

Eat snacks like dried fruit and nuts, which you can easily carry with you. Stay hydrated by drinking water, avoiding sugary drinks and alcohol, which can dehydrate you further.

7.4. Trying Local Cuisine

Local cuisines present an opportunity to explore and enjoy new flavors and textures, while also providing a cultural learning experience.

However, thorough research is paramount to ensure you're sampling local dishes that align with your dietary needs. Many regions have traditional dishes that are fresh, nutrient-dense, and flavorful.

Start your culinary exploration by trying small portions of various dishes. This allows you to taste a variety of foods without overeating. It's also vital to stay aware of any food allergies or intolerances you might have when trying new foods.

7.5. Opting for Self-Catering

Whenever possible, opt for accommodation like a serviced apartment or a hotel room with a small kitchenette. This allows you to prepare some meals yourself.

Visit local markets to buy fresh produce. Not only is this an excellent opportunity to get to know the local flavors, but it also allows you to control what goes in your food. Even simple meals like breakfast or a light dinner can make a significant difference in maintaining a healthy eating pattern.

7.6. Maintaining Hydration Levels

Hydration is as important as nutrition, especially when travelling. Dehydration can cause fatigue, impact brain function, and even confuse feelings of thirst for hunger, leading to overeating.

Aim to drink a minimum of 8-10 glasses of water each day. Increase your intake if you're traveling to a hot climate or partaking in physical activities such as hiking or trekking.

7.7. Healthy Eating while Sightseeing

When sightseeing, take along some nutritious snacks. Fresh fruits, nuts, seeds, or a small sandwich can be adequate for maintaining energy levels until it's time for a proper meal.

Avoid the temptation of street food, unless you know what goes into it. Also, most of these foods are often deep-fried or heavily seasoned.

Eating healthy while traveling does require a bit of planning, mindfulness, and often some compromise. But it's definitely possible, and surprisingly easier once you get the hang of it. Just remember, every meal doesn't have to be perfect; it's what we do consistently that counts the most to our health. So enjoy your travels, and make the journey as nourishing for your body as it is for your soul!

Chapter 8. Combating Jet Lag: Aligning Sleep and Exercise Routines

Jet lag deserves its reputation as one of the most notorious side effects of air travel, especially for those crossing multiple time zones. Its symptoms range from mild discomfort to debilitating fatigue and disorientation. While your watch might tell you it's mid-afternoon, your body's internal clock could still be set to the middle of the night - a discombobulating experience, to be sure. A proactive approach will not only help you combat jet lag but also set you up for success in maintaining your fitness routine while on the move.

8.1. Understanding Jet Lag and Its Impact on Fitness

Key to managing jet lag is understanding its root cause. In scientific terms, it is a physiological condition resulting from disturbances to an individual's circadian rhythms, also known as your "body clock." This biological cycle regulates a myriad of bodily functions, including sleep, digestion, cellular repair, and hormonal balance.

For fitness enthusiasts, jet lag's impact extends beyond mere feelings of tiredness; it can also take a toll on performance. When your circadian rhythm is disturbed, your body's ability to repair muscle tissue is compromised. Your appetite regulation might be off, causing unhealthful eating habits. This cascades into a suboptimal exercise routine and, if unchecked, could thwart your fitness goals.

8.2. Sleep Management Strategies: Foundation of Recovery

The relationship between good sleep and fitness is bi-directional: while adequate sleep supports physical performance, regular exercise can improve the quality of your sleep too. Thus, maintaining your training regimen while managing your sleep is crucial in mitigating jet lag.

+ **Adjust to your new sleep schedule gradually** Ease your body into its new schedule by gradually shifting your sleep and wake times to coincide with those of the new time zone.

+ **Sleep aids and supplements** Be cautious if you choose to use sleep aids. Some supplements such as melatonin can be effective, but you should consult your healthcare provider first to understand dosage and potential side effects.

+ **Consider light exposure** Light plays a vital role in regulating your biological clock. Avoid light when it's night in the destination pre-flight and seek sunshine whenever it's daytime there.

8.3. Fighting Jet-Lag with Nutrition

The food you consume can work with your body to better regulate your internal clock. Studies have shown that time-restrictive eating, where you eat according to the new time zone hours before your journey, can favorably influence your circadian rhythms.

Hydration can't be emphasized enough when traveling. Arid cabin air can lead to dehydration, which in turn exacerbates jet lag symptoms. Good hydration supports all your body's physiological functions, including the muscle recovery process after workouts.

8.4. Activating Your Body: Exercise to Conclude Jet Lag

Exercise can serve as a potent cure to shake off jet lag. However, be mindful of the type, the timing, and the intensity of your workouts.

+ **Type of exercise** Light cardio or body mobility exercises such as yoga or stretching can boost your alertness upon arriving at your destination.

+ **Timing of your workout** Avoid heavy workouts close to bedtime given their alerting effects. Plan more demanding sessions in the natural light of morning/early afternoon to help adjust your internal clock.

+ **Intensity of workouts** Wisely gauge exercise intensity. On the first day, choose more calming, low-impact workouts to soothe the body.

Using sleep and exercise, supported by good nutrition, you can turn the tables on jet lag. Despite the often complex nature of these strategies, with practice and adjustment to individual needs, they become invaluable tools in managing jet lag. Maintaining your normal exercise routine while traveling can be challenging, but not impossible in the face of jet lag. After all, the ultimate goal is to enjoy our travels while keeping our commitment to health and fitness intact. It may take a few trials to find what works best for you, but once you do, not only will your travels be more enjoyable, you will also maintain your fitness standards no matter the time zone.

Chapter 9. Hotel Room Workouts: Your Portable Gym

Even if your travels include upscale hotels with noteworthy gyms, there are times when an in-room workout is the most feasible option. We are unlocking the potential of your hotel room to transform into a makeshift gym, enabling you to maintain your fitness routine despite being on the move.

9.1. Hotel Furniture-as-Gym Equipment

Let's start the tour by repurposing the room furniture into your workout equipment.

Desk Chair: Perfect for tricep dips and inclined push-ups, the ubiquitous hotel room chair can become your upper body workout equipment.

Bed: Besides being a cozy place to sleep, the hotel bed can become a soft mat for abdominal workouts or stretches. It even doubles up as a supportive surface for resistance exercises like push-ups.

Suitcase: Wondering where to find weights in your hotel room? Look no further than your own suitcase. Packed bags can act as makeshift weights for a variety of arm and leg exercises.

9.2. The Perfect Hotel Room Workout Routine

Here is a step-by-step guide to a full-body workout routine using just your hotel room amenities.

1. Warm-Up: Start with 5-10 minutes of light cardio. A few rounds of high knees, jumping jacks, or even a brisk walk around your room should do the trick.

2. Upper Body: Use the chair for tricep dips and push-ups. For tricep dips, seat yourself on the edge of the chair and place your hands beside your hips. Slide your butt off, bending at the elbows to do the dips. For push-ups, place your hands on the chair's seat, extend your legs and lower your body towards the chair, then push yourself up.

3. Lower Body: Your suitcase is perfect for squats and lunges. Hold it like a kettlebell and descend into a squat, keeping your chest up and back straight. For lunges, stand straight, step one leg forward, lower your body until both knees are at 90 degrees, then push up through the front heel.

4. Core: Use the bed for a variety of core workouts. Do sit-ups by tucking your feet under the edge of the mattress for stability or planks by placing your forearms on the bed, extending your legs and holding the position.

5. Cool Down: End your workout with 5-10 minutes of stretching on the carpet or bed. This will help avoid muscle stiffness and promote recovery.

Repeat this routine as convenient and desired during your stay.

9.3. Nutrition Tips for Fitness Enthusiasts

Maintaining your diet is just as important as sticking to your workout routine. Here are a few tips to keep your nutrition in check while staying in a hotel.

1. Plan Ahead: Most hotels provide in-room dining menus online. Before you travel, check out the menu and plan your meals to include lots of vegetables, lean proteins, and complex carbohydrates.

2. Stay Hydrated: Travel often leads to dehydration. Keep a water bottle handy and refill it regularly.

3. Avoid Excessive Room Service: It's easy to overeat when opting for room service due to portion sizes typically being larger than necessary. Opt for healthier alternatives or split your meals.

Remember, consistency is the key. Irrespective of how fancy or modest your hotel room is, it has the potential to serve as your personal gym. Combine your in-room workouts with conscious nutrition choices for a comprehensive fitness strategy while traveling. This way, you'll never miss a workout or have to compromise on your diet, no matter where your travels take you.

And thus, the hotel room, often only thought of as a place of rest and relaxation, is transformed into a center for physical wellbeing. With these techniques in your travel toolkit, there's no destination that can deter your dedication to fitness. Broaden your fitness horizons and make every journey a step towards optimal health. After all, it's not just about reaching your destination, but also about enjoying the journey in the strongest, healthiest body possible.

Chapter 10. Supplements and Hydration: Keeping Fit While Flying

Contrary to popular belief, your journey to maintaining optimum fitness begins even before your flight is up in the air. The time you spend in transit adds up, which might cause substantial disruptions to your regular exercise and diet routines. However, two primary factors can make a monumental difference when you are jet-setting around - supplements and hydration. Armed with the right supplements and proper hydration routine, keeping fit while flying becomes a task that is not just possible, but surprisingly comfortable.

10.1. The Importance of Supplements for Travelers

While traveling, your body is exposed to a unique set of challenges. Different time zones, irregular sleep schedules, and changes in diet put your body's natural routine out of sync. Supplements can play a crucial role in helping mitigate these changes and ensure your body receives all the nutrients it needs.

10.1.1. Essential Supplements for Travel

There isn't a one-size-fits-all approach when it comes to choosing supplements for travel; what works best varies from person to person, and your regular diet should inform your choices. Nevertheless, some supplements can be particularly beneficial for travelers:

1. Multivitamins: A great 'insurance policy' against any potential nutritional deficiencies, especially when your diet might not be

as balanced as you'd like.

2. Magnesium: Known to aid in sleep and muscle recovery, Magnesium can be helpful when you're jet-setting across different time zones.

3. Probiotics: Long flights can wreak havoc on your gut health, which can further take a toll on your immune system. Probiotics can help maintain a healthy gut during these periods of potential stress.

4. Fish Oil: Rich in Omega-3 fatty acids that are essential for brain health, fish oil can aid in offsetting the mental fatigue that often accompanies travel.

Remember, always consult your doctor or a registered dietitian before adding any new supplement to your routine. Each person's needs are unique and understanding these will allow you to select the best supplement regimen for your lifestyle.

10.2. Supplement Dos and Don'ts

Regular supplementation can provide many health benefits. However, it's also essential to be aware of how and when to take them to optimize their effectiveness.

10.2.1. Key Dos to Remember

1. Do take your supplements with food: Most supplements, especially multivitamins and fish oil, are better absorbed when consumed with food.

2. Do pay attention to timing: Some supplements, like magnesium, work better at night as they can aid in relaxation and sleep.

3. Do stay flexible: If you miss a dose, don't panic. Just return to your routine as soon as you can.

10.2.2. Don'ts to Keep in Mind

1. Don't substitute supplements for a balanced diet: Supplements are there to top up your nutrition, not to replace meals. Aim to eat as healthily as possible.

2. Don't take more than recommended: More doesn't mean better in the world of supplements. Always stick to the recommended dosage.

Multi-dose travel containers are good for keeping your supplements organized. Sorting your supplements before traveling will not only save time but also ensure that you won't fall off track.

10.3. Hydration: A Must-Have for Every Traveler

The importance of hydration cannot be overstated, especially for those looking to stay fit while flying. The lack of humidity in the cabin air causes your body to lose water faster than usual, which can lead to symptoms like dry skin, fatigue, and headaches. While it is essential to hydrate, not all types of beverages are suitable for in-flight consumption.

10.3.1. Hydration Tips for Optimal Flight Fitness

Follow these hydration tips to help keep your body in prime condition during your flight:

1. Water is your best friend: Aim to drink at least 8-ounce glasses of water for every hour you're in the air.

2. Avoid caffeine and alcohol: Both these beverages can dehydrate your body further. Swap your coffee and wine for herbal teas or fresh fruit juice.

3. Add hydration-boosting foods to your travel snack pack:

Cucumbers, watermelon, and oranges are not just delicious but also high in water content.

10.4. Supplements and Hydration: Final Thoughts

It is widely thought that maintaining fitness while traveling is a monumental task. However, with thoughtful planning that includes supplement management and hydration, you can ensure your diet balances out and helps maintain your fitness routine while in the air. Take advantage of these tips to make your journey healthier, happier, and more fulfilling. After all, the journey is as important as the destination, and by caring for your body along the way, your travels can only be all the more enjoyable!

Chapter 11. Staying Motivated: App and Tech Support for Fitness Travelers

In the digital age, technology has made it extraordinarily easy to remain motivated, track progress, and optimize our fitness routines - especially while traveling. There's an extensive array of innovative apps and smart devices available that efface the challenges of maintaining a workout regimen or sticking to dietary plans during travel periods.

11.1. Get Moving with Fitness Apps

Fitness apps are specially optimized to keep you active and motivated. These health-based platforms offer structured workout regimes, track your activities, and provide insights about your performance.

1. **MyFitnessPal**: Renowned for its comprehensive food database, MyFitnessPal displays calories, nutrition facts, and a comprehensive journal of your consumption. It integrates with a variety of fitness apps and devices. Consider this app your personal dietitian on-the-go.

2. **7 Minute Workout**: For those always in a hurry, this app offers quick, effective, and no-equipment workouts. Just two or three tiny slots in your day, and you can contribute significantly to your health.

3. **Strava**: For outdoor enthusiasts, Strava efficiently tracks cycling and running workouts. Its social feature adds a competitive edge that can enhance motivation.

4. **Yoga Studio**: This app brings the serenity of yoga to your mobile

screen. It is perfect for tourists aiming to relax their minds while keeping bodies active.

5. **Workout Trainer**: Providing thousands of free workouts, Workout Trainer is the ultimate resource for fitness enthusiasts.

6. **FitStar Personal Trainer**: Personalization is key in FitStar. Workouts are created based on your ability and performance, and they get more challenging as you progress.

11.2. Step into the Smart era with Wearable Fitness Tech

Smart wearables have transformed the way travelers can track fitness. With these comfortable-to-wear gadgets, fitness data is literally at your fingertips.

1. **Fitbit**: Offering a variety of models, Fitbits track your daily steps, heart rate, sleep patterns, swimming workouts, distance traveled, calories burned, and active minutes.

2. **Apple Watch**: A trailblazer in health-based tech wearables, the Apple Watch moves beyond just activity tracking. It includes ECG, noise level, cycle tracking, and even fall detection.

3. **Garmin Vivoactive**: Renowned amongst the runners, cyclists, and swimmers, Garmin's GPS-enabled watches track a massive selection of sports.

4. **WHOOP Strap**: WHOOP Strap calculates your body strain from the day's workouts, stress, and sleep pattern. It offers daily recovery scores to understand when you are primed to push the body hard.

11.3. Use IoT for Functional Fitness Spaces

Internet of Things (IoT) can help convert your hotel room or Airbnb space into a functional workout zone. Connected fitness gear such as smart yoga mats, connected dumbbells, and more will ensure that you can maintain your workout routine regardless of where you are.

1. **Nexersys Boxing Unit**: Perfect for those who prefer HIIT workouts. It comes with personal profiles and real-time feedback.

2. **Tangram Smart Jump Rope**: This gadget measures your jump count, calories burned, and workout times. It also syncs with your smartphone to track your progress.

3. **Manduka Pro Smart Yoga Mat**: This yoga mat connects to your phone and gives you feedback on your balance and poses.

11.4. Harness the Power of Social Media

Online communities can also play a crucial part in maintaining your motivation. The prospect of sharing progress, or the sheer accountability from publicly posting goals, can provide the push needed to adhere to fitness routines.

Instagram, Facebook, and Twitter are platforms where you can find like-minded travelers, sharing experiences, tips, and advice all in real-time. Virtual challenges on platforms like 'My Virtual Mission' let you create a fitness mission and track it against others. Imagine running through your itinerary while still in your home country!

In conclusion, being away from home doesn't mean disconnecting from your fitness regimen. With smart tech and digital tools in the right place, you can make every travel journey an opportunity to improve health and fitness. In committing to a healthier lifestyle, even journeys around the world cannot distract you from your fitness goals. The best part? There are numerous options to choose from, guaranteeing that there is something for everyone.